CRYPTOSPORIDIOSIS RECOVERY COOKBOOK

Healing Recipes For Gut Health And Immunity Boost, Featuring Probiotic Meals And Nutrient-Rich Remedies

STEPHANIE LOUDER

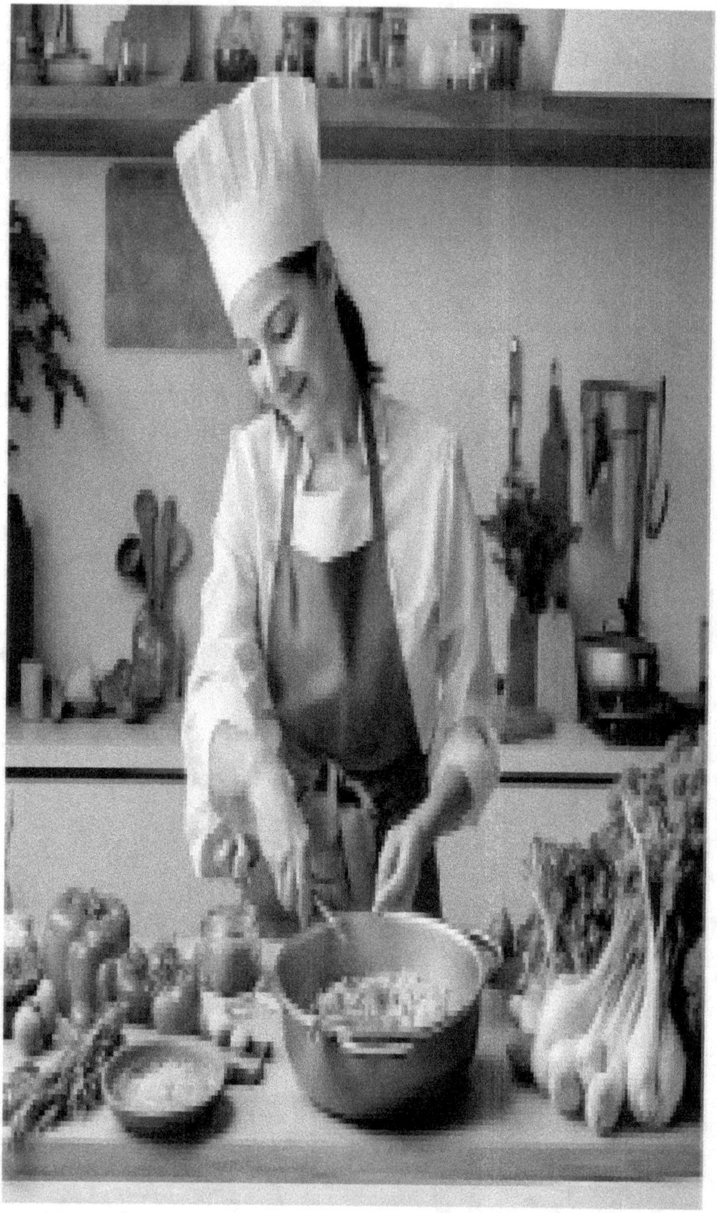

Contents

- CHAPTER 1 5
  - Introduction To Cryptosporidiosis Recovery 6
- CHAPTER 2 10
  - Breakfasts For Recovery 10
    - Energizing Smoothies and Juices 10
    - Nutrient-Packed Breakfast Bowls 11
    - Healing Porridges and Oatmeal Varieties 13
- CHAPTER 3 16
  - Wholesome Main Dishes 16
- CHAPTER 4 20
  - Brain-Boosting Salads And Dressings 20
    - Nutrient-Dense Salad Recipes 20
    - Homemade Dressing Varieties 22
- CHAPTER 5 25
  - Nourishing Soups And Stews 25
- CHAPTER 6 30
  - Memory-Enhancing Sandwiches And Wraps 30
    - Creative Sandwich Ideas: 30
    - Wraps for On-the-Go Nutrition: 33
- CHAPTER 7 37
  - Hydration And Brain-Boosting Beverages 37
- CHAPTER 8 41
  - Quick And Easy Recipes For Busy Days 41
- CHAPTER 9 46
  - Forbidden Foods And Substitutions 46

CHAPTER 10 52
  Desserts And Treats For Occasional Indulgence 52
CHAPTER 11 56
  Meal Plans And Customization 56
  Conclusion 61

Copyright © 2024 Stephanie Louder.

All rights reserved.

Unauthorized reproduction or distribution of this material is prohibited. For permissions, contact Stephanie Louder at stephanielouder13@gmail.com

Disclaimer

This book authored by Stephanie Louder, is provided for informational purposes only.

Neither the author nor the publisher assumes any responsibility for the use or misuse of the information herein. This guide does not endorse or support any specific platform or method. Readers are encouraged to consult with healthcare professionals for personalized advice.

CHAPTER 1
Introduction To Cryptosporidiosis Recovery

Cryptosporidiosis is a gastrointestinal illness caused by the parasite Cryptosporidium. It is commonly transmitted through contaminated water or food, and it can also spread through contact with infected animals or people.

The symptoms of cryptosporidiosis can range from mild diarrhea to severe dehydration, especially in vulnerable populations such as young children, elderly individuals, and those with weakened immune systems. Recovery from cryptosporidiosis involves not only medical treatment but also a focus on nutrition to support the body's healing process.

Understanding Cryptosporidiosis involves recognizing the nature of the infection and how it affects the digestive system. Cryptosporidium is a microscopic parasite that can cause diarrhea, stomach cramps, nausea, and vomiting.

It can be challenging to diagnose and treat, especially in cases where the immune system is compromised. Understanding the life cycle of the parasite and its impact on the body's ability to absorb nutrients is crucial for effective management and recovery.

The Importance of Nutrition in Recovery from cryptosporidiosis cannot be overstated. A well-balanced diet plays a vital role in supporting the immune system, replenishing lost nutrients, and restoring gut health.

Since cryptosporidiosis often leads to diarrhea and nutrient malabsorption, patients may experience deficiencies in essential vitamins and minerals. Therefore, nutrition becomes a cornerstone of treatment to aid in recovery and prevent complications.

Key Nutrients for Cryptosporidiosis Patients include those that support immune function, promote gut healing, and replenish electrolytes lost through diarrhea.

Vitamin A is crucial for maintaining mucosal integrity in the gut and supporting immune responses. Zinc is another essential nutrient that aids in immune function and wound healing. Electrolytes such as potassium, sodium, and magnesium are vital for hydration and maintaining electrolyte balance, especially during episodes of diarrhea.

Foods to Include in a Cryptosporidiosis Recovery Diet are those that are easy to digest, rich in nutrients, and gentle on the stomach. Bland foods like rice, boiled potatoes, and cooked vegetables can provide essential nutrients without exacerbating digestive symptoms.

Lean proteins such as chicken, fish, and tofu can help rebuild muscle tissue and support overall recovery. Incorporating probiotic-rich foods like yogurt and kefir can also promote a healthy gut microbiome and aid in digestion.

On the other hand, Foods to Avoid during cryptosporidiosis recovery are those that are difficult to digest or may irritate the digestive system. Spicy foods, high-fat foods, and excessive caffeine or alcohol can worsen symptoms such as diarrhea and stomach cramps. Foods that are known allergens or intolerances should also be avoided to prevent further gastrointestinal distress.

Recovery from cryptosporidiosis requires a holistic approach that includes medical treatment, proper hydration, and a nutrient-dense diet. Understanding the nature of the infection, the importance of nutrition in healing, key nutrients for support, and foods to include and avoid can significantly improve outcomes and promote a speedy recovery for patients affected by cryptosporidiosis.

CHAPTER 2
Breakfasts For Recovery

Energizing Smoothies and Juices

Energizing smoothies and juices are excellent choices for a nutritious and revitalizing start to your day, especially during a recovery period.

These beverages are packed with vitamins, minerals, antioxidants, and other essential nutrients that can support your body's healing process.

When crafting energizing smoothies, consider incorporating a variety of fruits such as berries, bananas, mangoes, and citrus fruits like oranges or grapefruits. These fruits are rich in vitamin C, which boosts immunity and aids in tissue repair. Additionally, adding leafy greens like spinach or kale provides a dose of fiber, vitamins A, K, and folate, contributing to overall wellness.

To enhance the protein content of your smoothies, consider including ingredients like

Greek yogurt, almond milk, or plant-based protein powders. Protein is crucial for muscle repair and regeneration, making it essential during recovery from illness or injury.

Incorporating healthy fats into your smoothies can further enhance their nutritional value. Ingredients like avocado, chia seeds, or flaxseeds provide omega-3 fatty acids, which have anti-inflammatory properties and support brain health.

When it comes to energizing juices, opt for freshly squeezed varieties to maximize nutrient intake.

A combination of fruits and vegetables, such as carrots, apples, ginger, and beets, can create a flavorful and nutrient-rich juice. Be mindful of added sugars in store-bought juices and opt for homemade versions or those with no added sugars.

Nutrient-Packed Breakfast Bowls

Nutrient-packed breakfast bowls offer a customizable and wholesome option for starting your day on the right nutritional note.

These bowls typically consist of a base, such as oats, quinoa, or Greek yogurt, layered with a variety of nutrient-dense toppings.

Oats, whether in the form of rolled oats, steel-cut oats, or oat bran, are a versatile and fiber-rich base for breakfast bowls. They provide sustained energy, promote digestive health, and can be paired with a range of toppings to suit individual preferences.

For protein-rich breakfast bowls, consider adding ingredients like nuts (almonds, walnuts), seeds (chia seeds, pumpkin seeds), or nut butters (almond butter, peanut butter). Greek yogurt is another excellent source of protein and can serve as a creamy base for your bowl.

Incorporating fresh or frozen fruits into your breakfast bowl adds natural sweetness, vitamins, and antioxidants. Berries, sliced bananas, diced apples, and tropical fruits like pineapple or mango can all complement the flavors and textures of your bowl.

To add crunch and additional nutrients, consider including toppings like granola (preferably low in added sugars), toasted coconut flakes, cacao nibs, or crushed nuts/seeds. These toppings not only enhance the taste but also provide essential nutrients like fiber, healthy fats, and micronutrients.

Drizzling a small amount of honey, maple syrup, or a dollop of natural fruit preserves can add a touch of sweetness without overwhelming the nutritional balance of your breakfast bowl.

Healing Porridges and Oatmeal Varieties

Healing porridges and oatmeal varieties offer comfort and nourishment, making them ideal choices for individuals focusing on recovery. These warm and hearty dishes can be customized with a range of ingredients to support overall well-being.

Traditional oatmeal, cooked with water or milk (dairy or plant-based), serves as a blank canvas for adding nutritious elements. Consider incorporating spices like cinnamon, nutmeg, or ginger for added flavor and potential health benefits, such as anti-inflammatory properties.

For added protein and creaminess, stir in a scoop of protein powder (vanilla or unflavored) or a spoonful of Greek yogurt into your oatmeal. This addition not only enhances the texture but also provides a satiating boost of protein.

To boost the fiber content of your porridge, add ingredients like ground flaxseeds, chia seeds, or hemp hearts. These superfoods contribute to digestive health, heart health, and overall wellness.

Incorporating fruits into your porridge can elevate both the taste and nutritional profile. Fresh fruits like sliced bananas, berries, diced apples, or cooked fruits like stewed peaches or pears add natural sweetness, vitamins, and antioxidants.

For those with dietary preferences or restrictions, exploring alternative grain options can provide variety and additional nutrients. Consider using quinoa, amaranth, buckwheat, or millet as bases for your healing porridge, each offering unique flavors and nutritional benefits.

To add a final touch of indulgence and nutrient density, consider garnishing your porridge with a sprinkle of toasted nuts/seeds, a drizzle of almond or coconut butter, or a dash of pure vanilla extract. These additions enhance the overall sensory experience while contributing to a balanced and nourishing breakfast.

CHAPTER 3
Wholesome Main Dishes

Wholesome Main Dishes play a crucial role in supporting recovery and overall well-being, especially for individuals focusing on improving their health. Within this realm, there are several key concepts that contribute to creating nourishing and satisfying meals: Lean Protein Options for Recovery, Healing Grains and Legumes, and Vegetable-Centric Main Courses.

Lean Protein Options for Recovery are essential components of a balanced meal plan, particularly for those undergoing recovery or dealing with health challenges. These proteins are typically low in saturated fats and cholesterol, making them heart-friendly choices. Examples of lean proteins include skinless poultry, such as chicken or turkey breast, lean cuts of beef or pork, tofu, tempeh, and legumes like lentils, chickpeas, and beans. Incorporating lean proteins into main dishes provides the body with essential amino acids necessary for tissue repair and muscle recovery, supporting overall healing.

Healing Grains and Legumes are rich in nutrients like fiber, vitamins, and minerals, making them valuable additions to main dishes for recovery. Whole grains such as quinoa, brown rice, barley, and whole wheat provide sustained energy and promote digestive health.

Legumes, including beans, peas, and lentils, are excellent plant-based protein sources that also contribute to heart health and blood sugar regulation. Combining healing grains and legumes in main dishes not only enhances nutritional value but also adds texture and flavor diversity, making meals more enjoyable and satisfying.

Vegetable-Centric Main Courses emphasize the importance of incorporating a variety of vegetables into main dishes for their nutritional benefits and culinary versatility. Vegetables are rich in vitamins, minerals, antioxidants, and fiber, supporting immune function, digestion, and overall health. Including a colorful array of vegetables such as leafy greens, cruciferous vegetables like broccoli and Brussels sprouts, root vegetables like carrots and sweet potatoes, and colorful bell peppers and tomatoes ensures a well-rounded meal that promotes healing and recovery.

Vegetable-centric main courses can include stir-fries, salads, roasted vegetable platters, and vegetable-based stews or curries, offering endless possibilities for nutritious and delicious meals.

When creating wholesome main dishes, it's important to consider the balance of macronutrients (proteins, carbohydrates, and fats) and micronutrients (vitamins and minerals) to support recovery and overall wellness. Incorporating lean protein options ensures adequate protein intake for tissue repair and immune function, while healing grains and legumes provide essential nutrients and sustained energy. Vegetable-centric main courses not only add nutritional value but also contribute to the flavor, texture, and visual appeal of meals, making them more enjoyable and satisfying.

By focusing on these key concepts, individuals can create nourishing main dishes that support their recovery journey and promote long-term health and well-being.

CHAPTER 4
Brain-Boosting Salads And Dressings

Salads have long been touted as a healthy choice for meals, but when crafted with a focus on brain health, they can become powerful tools for cognitive well-being.

The concept of brain-boosting salads goes beyond mere nutrition; it encompasses a thoughtful combination of ingredients that are known for their cognitive benefits. These salads are designed not just to satiate hunger but to nourish and support the brain's functions, from enhancing memory to promoting mental clarity and focus.

Nutrient-Dense Salad Recipes

Creating nutrient-dense salads involves selecting ingredients that are rich in vitamins, minerals, antioxidants, and other compounds known to support brain health. Dark leafy greens such as kale, spinach, and arugula are staples in these salads, providing essential nutrients like folate, vitamin K, and antioxidants that protect brain cells from oxidative stress. Including a variety of colorful vegetables like bell peppers, tomatoes, carrots, and broccoli adds a spectrum of vitamins, minerals, and phytonutrients crucial for optimal brain function.

Incorporating healthy fats is another key aspect of nutrient-dense salads. Avocado, known for its monounsaturated fats and vitamin E content, not only adds creaminess but also supports brain health by reducing inflammation and protecting cells. Nuts and seeds such as walnuts, almonds, flaxseeds, and chia seeds contribute omega-3 fatty acids, which are essential for cognitive function and can improve memory and concentration.

Protein plays a vital role in brain-boosting salads as well. Lean sources of protein like grilled chicken, tofu, chickpeas, or quinoa not only add texture and flavor but also provide amino acids necessary for neurotransmitter production. Including protein in salads helps maintain stable blood sugar levels and supports overall brain health and mood regulation.

To enhance the nutritional profile of these salads further, incorporating superfoods like berries, pomegranate seeds, and spirulina can add a potent dose of antioxidants, vitamins, and minerals. These ingredients not only contribute to the salad's visual appeal but also boost its brain-boosting properties, protecting against cognitive decline and supporting neuroplasticity.

Homemade Dressing Varieties

Pairing nutrient-dense salads with homemade dressings not only elevates their flavors but also ensures they remain healthy and free from additives often found in store-bought dressings. Creating homemade dressings allows for customization based on flavor preferences while incorporating ingredients that offer additional nutritional benefits.

A simple vinaigrette made with extra-virgin olive oil, balsamic vinegar, Dijon mustard, garlic, and a touch of honey or maple syrup not only adds tanginess to salads but also provides healthy fats, antioxidants, and anti-inflammatory properties. Olive oil, in particular, is rich in monounsaturated fats and polyphenols that support brain health and reduce the risk of cognitive decline.

Creamy dressings can be made healthier by using Greek yogurt or avocado as a base instead of mayonnaise or heavy cream. A Greek yogurt-based dressing flavored with herbs like dill, parsley, or cilantro not only adds creaminess but also contributes probiotics beneficial for gut health, which in turn can impact brain function through the gut-brain axis.

Incorporating herbs and spices into dressings not only enhances flavor but also adds nutritional value. Turmeric, known for its anti-inflammatory and antioxidant properties due to curcumin, can be added to dressings for a vibrant color and brain-protective benefits. Fresh herbs like basil, mint, and rosemary not only lend freshness but also offer additional antioxidants and phytonutrients.

Experimenting with citrus-based dressings using lemon, lime, or orange juice adds a refreshing acidity while providing vitamin C and flavonoids that support brain health and reduce oxidative stress. Combining citrus with olive oil, herbs, and a touch of honey or mustard creates a balanced and flavorful dressing that complements brain-boosting salads perfectly.

Overall, the concept of homemade dressings for brain-boosting salads revolves around using wholesome ingredients that contribute to overall health while enhancing the flavors and nutritional benefits of salads. By incorporating a variety of nutrient-dense ingredients and experimenting with different dressing combinations, these salads become not just a meal but a nourishing experience that supports cognitive function and well-being.

CHAPTER 5
Nourishing Soups And Stews

Nourishing Soups and Stews play a significant role in supporting overall health and well-being, particularly during times of recovery and when aiming to boost the immune system.

These culinary creations are not just meals; they are comforting, nutrient-dense, and often therapeutic in nature. Immune-Boosting Soup Recipes are crafted with ingredients known for their immune-boosting properties, such as antioxidants, vitamins, and minerals that help strengthen the body's defense mechanisms. These soups are designed to provide a flavorful and nourishing experience while aiding in the body's natural ability to fight off illnesses and recover from various health challenges.

One of the key aspects of Immune-Boosting Soup Recipes is the careful selection of ingredients. These soups often include a variety of vegetables, herbs, and spices known for their immune-boosting properties.

For example, ingredients like garlic, ginger, turmeric, and leafy greens are commonly used due to their antibacterial, anti-inflammatory, and antioxidant properties. These ingredients not only add depth of flavor to the soups but also contribute to their healing and immune-supportive qualities.

Additionally, Immune-Boosting Soup Recipes may incorporate protein sources such as lean meats, poultry, or plant-based proteins like beans and lentils. Protein is essential for supporting the immune system and aiding in the repair and regeneration of tissues, making it an important component of recovery-focused soups. Moreover, incorporating healthy fats like olive oil or avocado into these soups can further enhance their nutritional value and contribute to overall well-being.

The cooking methods used in preparing Immune-Boosting Soup Recipes also contribute to their health benefits.

Slow cooking or simmering ingredients allows flavors to meld together while preserving nutrients. This gentle cooking process helps retain the integrity of vitamins and minerals, ensuring that the soups deliver maximum nourishment.

In contrast, Comforting Stews for Recovery offer a different culinary experience focused on warmth, heartiness, and comfort. These stews are often characterized by their rich flavors and hearty textures, making them satisfying meals that can aid in recovery by providing essential nutrients and comforting the body and mind.

The ingredients chosen for Comforting Stews for Recovery are selected not only for their nutritional value but also for their ability to create a sense of comfort and well-being.

Root vegetables like carrots, potatoes, and parsnips are commonly found in Comforting Stews for Recovery, adding sweetness and substance to the dishes. These vegetables are rich in vitamins, minerals, and fiber, promoting digestive health and providing a steady source of energy. Additionally, stews may feature lean cuts of meat or plant-based proteins like tempeh or tofu, adding protein to support muscle recovery and overall strength.

Herbs and spices play a crucial role in enhancing the flavors of Comforting Stews for Recovery. Ingredients such as thyme, rosemary, and bay leaves add depth and complexity to the stews while offering potential health benefits such as anti-inflammatory and antioxidant properties. Warm spices like cinnamon and nutmeg may also be used to impart a comforting aroma and flavor profile to the stews.

The cooking process for Comforting Stews for Recovery often involves slow simmering or braising, allowing the ingredients to meld together and develop rich flavors. This slow cooking method not only enhances the taste of the stews but also helps break down tough cuts of meat or root vegetables, resulting in tender and flavorful dishes that are easy to digest.

Overall, Nourishing Soups and Stews, whether focused on immune-boosting properties or comforting qualities for recovery, offer a holistic approach to nourishing the body and supporting overall well-being.

By carefully selecting ingredients, incorporating essential nutrients, and utilizing gentle cooking methods, these culinary creations provide not only sustenance but also comfort and healing during times of recovery and beyond.

CHAPTER 6
Memory-Enhancing Sandwiches And Wraps

When it comes to crafting memory-enhancing sandwiches and wraps, creativity plays a vital role in not just satisfying hunger but also nourishing the brain. These culinary creations can be more than just a convenient meal; they can be a powerhouse of nutrients designed to boost cognitive function and support overall brain health. Let's delve into the concepts of memory-enhancing sandwiches and wraps, exploring creative ideas for both and highlighting their significance in providing on-the-go nutrition.

Creative Sandwich Ideas:

1.   Brain-Boosting Fillings: The foundation of a memory-enhancing sandwich lies in its fillings. Incorporating ingredients rich in omega-3 fatty acids, such as salmon or walnuts, can support brain function and memory retention. Avocado, known for its healthy fats and antioxidants, can

also be a star player in these sandwiches. Additionally, including leafy greens like spinach or kale provides essential vitamins and minerals, further enhancing the nutritional value.

2. Whole Grain Goodness: Opting for whole grain bread or wraps adds an extra layer of nutritional benefit. Whole grains are a great source of fiber, which aids in maintaining stable blood sugar levels and promotes better cognitive performance. They also contain B vitamins, essential for brain health and energy production. Experimenting with different types of whole grain bread, such as multigrain or sprouted grain, can add variety and texture to the sandwiches.

3. Antioxidant-Rich Additions: Adding fruits like blueberries, strawberries, or sliced apples not only adds sweetness and crunch but also introduces powerful antioxidants into the mix. Antioxidants help combat oxidative stress in the brain, potentially reducing the risk of cognitive decline. Incorporating a spread made from antioxidant-rich ingredients like hummus, roasted

red peppers, or beetroot can further elevate the sandwich's nutritional profile.

4. Protein-Packed Options: Including lean proteins such as grilled chicken, turkey, tofu, or hard-boiled eggs ensures a satisfying and balanced sandwich. Protein is essential for neurotransmitter function and can help improve concentration and memory. Consider marinating proteins with herbs and spices like rosemary, turmeric, or garlic, which have brain-boosting properties and add flavor complexity to the sandwich.

5. Healthy Fats for Flavor: Incorporating healthy fats like olive oil, nut butters, or a sprinkle of seeds (such as flaxseeds or chia seeds) not only enhances flavor but also provides essential fatty acids crucial for brain health.

These fats support neuronal communication and help maintain the integrity of cell membranes, promoting optimal cognitive function.

6. Herbs and Spices for a Flavorful Punch: Experimenting with herbs and spices can take a sandwich from ordinary to extraordinary. Fresh herbs like basil, cilantro, or mint not only add freshness but also contribute phytonutrients with potential cognitive benefits. Spices such as cinnamon, turmeric, or cumin not only add depth of flavor but also offer anti-inflammatory properties that can benefit brain health.

Wraps for On-the-Go Nutrition:
Wraps offer a convenient and portable way to enjoy a nutrient-dense meal, making them ideal for on-the-go nutrition. Here are some concepts to consider when creating memory-enhancing wraps:

1. Variety of Wraps: Explore different types of wraps beyond traditional flour tortillas, such as whole wheat, spinach, or even gluten-free options for those with dietary restrictions. These variations not only offer diverse flavors but also introduce additional nutrients into the meal.

2. Colorful and Nutrient-Rich Fillings: Similar to sandwiches, wraps benefit from a colorful array of fillings.

Incorporate a mix of vegetables like bell peppers, cucumbers, shredded carrots, and leafy greens to provide vitamins, minerals, and antioxidants. Adding a source of lean protein, whether grilled chicken, chickpeas, or grilled tofu, ensures satiety and supports muscle and brain function.

3. Innovative Spreads and Sauces: The spread or sauce used in a wrap can significantly impact its flavor and nutritional profile.

Consider options like yogurt-based dressings, tahini sauce, or avocado spreads for creaminess and added nutrients. These additions not only enhance the wrap's taste but also contribute healthy fats and essential nutrients.

4. Texture and Crunch: Incorporating elements that add texture and crunch, such as roasted nuts, seeds, or crispy vegetables like

jicama or radishes, can make the wrap more satisfying and enjoyable to eat.

Texture variation also adds a sensory aspect to the meal, enhancing the overall dining experience.

5. Balance of Flavors: Aim for a balance of flavors in wraps, combining sweet, savory, tangy, and spicy elements. This balance not only makes the wrap more interesting but also stimulates the palate and encourages mindful eating. Consider using ingredients like dried fruits, pickled vegetables, fresh herbs, or a dash of citrus for flavor complexity.

6. Portability and Convenience: One of the key advantages of wraps is their portability. Wraps can be tightly rolled and packed for easy transport, making them an excellent choice for busy days or meals on the move. Preparing wraps ahead of time and wrapping them in parchment paper or foil helps maintain their

freshness and structural integrity until ready to eat.

By incorporating these creative ideas into memory-enhancing sandwiches and wraps, you can not only enjoy delicious and satisfying meals but also nourish your brain with a range of nutrients that support cognitive function, memory retention, and overall well-being.

Experimenting with different ingredients, flavors, and textures allows for endless possibilities, ensuring that each wrap or sandwich is a delightful culinary experience packed with brain-boosting benefits.

CHAPTER 7
Hydration And Brain-Boosting Beverages

Hydration is a fundamental aspect of overall health and plays a crucial role in recovery from various illnesses and conditions. In the context of recovery, hydration refers to maintaining an optimal balance of fluids in the body to support physiological functions, promote healing, and enhance overall well-being.

This balance is especially vital for patients recovering from illnesses like Alzheimer's Disease, where hydration can directly impact cognitive function and overall recovery outcomes.

The importance of hydration for recovery cannot be overstated. Water is essential for numerous bodily functions, including maintaining proper cell function, regulating body temperature, aiding digestion, and flushing out toxins. During recovery, adequate hydration is critical for supporting the immune system, optimizing nutrient absorption, and promoting tissue repair and regeneration. Dehydration, on the other hand, can lead to a range of complications, including fatigue, impaired cognitive function, muscle cramps, and delayed healing processes.

For patients recovering from Alzheimer's Disease or other cognitive conditions, maintaining proper hydration levels is particularly crucial. Studies have shown that even mild dehydration can negatively impact cognitive performance, including memory, attention, and executive function. In older adults, dehydration can exacerbate cognitive decline and increase the risk of delirium and other complications.

In addition to water, certain brain-boosting beverages can play a role in supporting cognitive function and enhancing recovery outcomes.

These beverages are often rich in nutrients, antioxidants, and compounds that have been linked to brain health and cognitive performance. Incorporating brain-boosting beverages into a recovery diet can complement hydration efforts and provide additional benefits for patients undergoing rehabilitation or recovery from neurological conditions.

Brain-enhancing drink recipes can be tailored to include ingredients that are known for their cognitive benefits. For example, beverages infused with herbal teas like green tea or chamomile can provide antioxidants and compounds that support brain function and reduce inflammation. Smoothies and shakes made with ingredients such as berries, spinach, avocado, and nuts can offer a combination of vitamins, minerals, healthy fats, and phytonutrients that nourish the brain and promote neuronal health.

Certain beverages, such as coconut water or electrolyte-rich drinks, can also help replenish electrolytes lost during sweating or illness, supporting hydration and overall recovery. Adding natural sweeteners like honey or maple syrup can enhance flavor while providing energy-boosting benefits. Incorporating ingredients like turmeric, ginger, and cinnamon can add anti-inflammatory properties and enhance the nutritional profile of brain-boosting beverages.

The key to creating effective brain-enhancing drink recipes lies in selecting nutrient-dense ingredients that support cognitive function and overall health. These beverages should be hydrating, nourishing, and enjoyable to encourage regular consumption and support long-term recovery goals. By including a variety of brain-boosting beverages in a recovery diet, patients can enhance hydration, promote brain health, and optimize their journey toward recovery and improved well-being.

CHAPTER 8
Quick And Easy Recipes For Busy Days

Creating quick and easy recipes for busy days is a practical approach to maintaining a healthy diet and managing time efficiently. Whether you're a working professional, a busy parent, or someone with a hectic schedule, having simple meal options can make a significant difference in maintaining a balanced diet without compromising on nutrition.

When it comes to quick and easy recipes, simplicity is key. These recipes often involve minimal ingredients, straightforward cooking techniques, and short preparation times. The goal is to streamline the cooking process without sacrificing flavor or nutritional value. One of the essential aspects of these recipes is their adaptability—they can be adjusted based on dietary preferences, allergies, or ingredient availability.

A common theme in quick and easy recipes is the use of fresh and wholesome ingredients.

While convenience foods have their place in a busy lifestyle, incorporating whole foods like fruits, vegetables, lean proteins, whole grains, and healthy fats ensures that the meals are nutritious and satisfying. Additionally, using herbs, spices, and simple homemade sauces can elevate the flavors of these dishes without adding complexity.

Simple meals for limited time and energy are designed to be accessible to anyone, regardless of their cooking experience. These meals often involve basic cooking techniques such as sautéing, roasting, boiling, or grilling.

The focus is on creating dishes that are easy to prepare, require minimal cleanup, and can be made in a short amount of time.

Batch cooking and meal prep are valuable strategies for busy individuals looking to save time and streamline their meal planning. Batch cooking involves preparing larger quantities of food at once, which can then be portioned and stored for future meals.

This approach is especially useful for staples like grains, proteins, soups, and stews. Meal prep involves preparing components of meals in advance, such as chopping vegetables, marinating proteins, or assembling salads. Having these prepped ingredients on hand makes it easier to throw together a quick and nutritious meal during busy times.

When creating quick and easy recipes, it's important to consider nutritional balance. Meals should include a mix of macronutrients (carbohydrates, proteins, and fats), as well as micronutrients (vitamins and minerals). Incorporating a variety of colors and textures not only makes the meals visually appealing but also ensures a diverse range of nutrients.

For example, a quick and easy meal idea could be a quinoa salad with roasted vegetables and grilled chicken. To prepare this dish, cook quinoa according to package instructions and let it cool. Meanwhile, toss chopped vegetables (such as bell peppers, zucchini, and cherry tomatoes) with olive oil, salt, and pepper, then roast them in the oven until tender. Grill chicken breasts seasoned with herbs and spices until cooked through.

To assemble the salad, combine the cooked quinoa, roasted vegetables, and sliced chicken. Drizzle with a simple vinaigrette made from olive oil, balsamic vinegar, Dijon mustard, and honey. Garnish with fresh herbs like parsley or basil for added flavor.

Another quick meal option is a stir-fry with tofu or shrimp and a variety of colorful vegetables. Simply sauté diced tofu or shrimp with garlic, ginger, and soy sauce until cooked. Add in chopped vegetables such as broccoli, carrots, and snap peas, and stir-fry until tender-crisp. Serve over cooked brown rice or quinoa for a complete and satisfying meal.

quick and easy recipes for busy days prioritize simplicity, freshness, and nutrition.

By incorporating whole foods, basic cooking techniques, and strategic meal planning strategies like batch cooking and meal prep, it's possible to enjoy delicious and healthy meals even during the busiest of times. These recipes empower individuals to take control of their diet and wellness without compromising on taste or convenience.

CHAPTER 9
Forbidden Foods And Substitutions

Understanding which foods to avoid during recovery is crucial for maintaining optimal health and supporting the healing process. Certain foods can hinder recovery by exacerbating symptoms, interfering with medication effectiveness, or causing digestive issues. By identifying and eliminating these forbidden foods, individuals can create a supportive dietary environment that promotes faster healing and overall well-being.

One category of forbidden foods during recovery includes processed and refined products. These often contain additives, preservatives, and artificial ingredients that can be harsh on the digestive system and may contribute to inflammation. Examples of such foods include processed meats like sausages and deli meats, sugary snacks and desserts, refined grains like white bread and pastries, and packaged convenience foods with high sodium content.

These foods can negatively impact energy levels, immune function, and overall recovery progress.

Additionally, foods high in trans fats and unhealthy fats should be avoided during recovery.

These fats, commonly found in fried foods, fast food items, and commercially baked goods, can increase inflammation in the body and impair cardiovascular health. Limiting or eliminating foods like fried chicken, potato chips, doughnuts, and commercial baked goods can support a healthier recovery diet.

Another group of forbidden foods includes those that are high in sugar and artificial sweeteners. Excessive sugar intake can lead to fluctuations in blood sugar levels, which may negatively affect energy levels, mood, and immune function. Artificial sweeteners, commonly found in diet sodas, sugar-free candies, and certain packaged foods, can also disrupt gut health and may contribute to digestive discomfort. Avoiding foods and beverages with added sugars and artificial sweeteners can help stabilize blood sugar levels and support overall recovery.

Inflammatory foods such as refined carbohydrates, processed oils, and high-glycemic index foods should also be restricted during recovery. These foods can contribute to inflammation in the body, which may worsen symptoms and delay healing. Examples of inflammatory foods to avoid include white rice, sugary drinks, vegetable oils high in omega-6 fatty acids (e.g., soybean oil, corn oil), and processed snacks like chips and crackers. Choosing whole grains, healthy fats (such as olive oil and avocado), and nutrient-dense snacks can help reduce inflammation and support recovery.

Moreover, individuals undergoing recovery should steer clear of allergenic foods that may trigger adverse reactions. Common allergens include gluten-containing grains (wheat, barley, rye), dairy products, nuts, shellfish, and eggs. For individuals with known food allergies or sensitivities, avoiding these allergenic foods is essential to prevent allergic reactions and promote optimal healing.

In terms of safe substitutes for restricted ingredients, there are numerous options available to accommodate dietary restrictions and support recovery goals. For example, individuals avoiding processed meats can opt for lean protein sources such as grilled chicken, fish, legumes, and tofu. These alternatives provide essential nutrients like protein, vitamins, and minerals without the added preservatives and unhealthy fats found in processed meats.

For those limiting sugar and artificial sweeteners, natural sweeteners like honey, maple syrup, and stevia can be used in moderation to add sweetness to dishes and beverages. These natural sweeteners offer a more wholesome alternative to refined sugars and artificial additives. Similarly, whole fruits can be incorporated into desserts and snacks to satisfy sweet cravings while providing fiber, vitamins, and antioxidants.

To replace inflammatory foods with healthier options, individuals can focus on whole, unprocessed foods that are rich in nutrients and beneficial compounds.

For instance, swapping refined grains with whole grains like quinoa, brown rice, and oats can increase fiber intake and support digestive health. Choosing healthy fats from sources like avocados, nuts, seeds, and olive oil can provide essential fatty acids and anti-inflammatory properties.

For allergenic foods, individuals can explore allergen-free alternatives that mimic the taste and texture of common allergens. For example, dairy-free milk alternatives (e.g., almond milk, coconut milk, oat milk) can be used in place of cow's milk in recipes and beverages. Gluten-free grains such as rice, corn, quinoa, and buckwheat can replace wheat-based products in meals like pasta, bread, and baked goods.

understanding forbidden foods and their safe substitutions is key to creating a supportive and nourishing diet during recovery. By avoiding processed and inflammatory foods, limiting sugar and artificial additives, and accommodating allergenic restrictions with suitable substitutes, individuals can optimize their nutritional intake and enhance the healing process. It's important to consult with a healthcare professional or registered dietitian to personalize dietary recommendations based on individual health needs and recovery goals.

CHAPTER 10
Desserts And Treats For Occasional Indulgence

Creating desserts and treats that are both indulgent and healthy can be a delightful culinary adventure, striking a balance between satisfying cravings and supporting overall well-being. When it comes to crafting these delectable delights, a key concept to embrace is the notion of healthier alternatives that still provide a satisfying experience. This involves incorporating nutrient-dense ingredients, reducing added sugars and unhealthy fats, and exploring innovative cooking techniques to enhance flavors without compromising on health.

One of the fundamental aspects of designing healthier desserts is the careful selection of ingredients. Instead of relying solely on refined sugars, which can contribute to health issues like diabetes and obesity, opting for natural sweeteners such as honey, maple syrup, or dates can add sweetness while offering nutritional benefits. These alternatives often contain vitamins, minerals, and antioxidants, making them a preferable choice for those looking to indulge without guilt. Additionally, using whole-grain flours or alternative flours like almond flour or coconut flour can boost fiber content and add a nutty richness to desserts.

Incorporating fruits into desserts is another strategy for adding natural sweetness and nutrition. Fresh fruits like berries, mangoes, and bananas not only lend a burst of flavor but also contribute vitamins, fiber, and antioxidants to the treats. From fruit salads and compotes to baked fruit crisps and sorbets, there are myriad ways to showcase the natural sweetness of fruits while keeping desserts light and refreshing. Furthermore, using unsweetened applesauce or mashed ripe bananas as binders or sweeteners in recipes can reduce the need for added sugars while adding moisture and texture.

When it comes to fats, choosing healthier options like plant-based fats (e.g., avocado, coconut oil) or small amounts of high-quality dairy can improve the nutritional profile of desserts. These fats can add creaminess and richness without the saturated fat content found in traditional butter or lard. Incorporating nuts and seeds, such as almonds, walnuts, or chia seeds, not only enhances texture but also provides healthy fats, protein, and essential nutrients.

Another crucial aspect of creating healthier desserts is mindful portion control and moderation. While it's tempting to indulge in large servings of decadent treats, practicing moderation allows for enjoying the flavors without overloading on calories and sugars. Portioning desserts into smaller servings, such as mini cupcakes, bite-sized bars, or individual parfaits, encourages mindful eating and prevents excessive consumption. Pairing desserts with protein or fiber-rich foods can also help balance blood sugar levels and promote satiety, reducing the temptation to overindulge.

Furthermore, exploring innovative cooking techniques can elevate the health quotient of desserts. Baking, grilling, or poaching fruits instead of frying or using excessive amounts of butter can retain their natural flavors and nutrients while reducing added fats. Incorporating herbs and spices like cinnamon, nutmeg, or vanilla not only enhances the taste but also adds antioxidants and anti-inflammatory properties to the desserts.

In essence, the concept of healthier alternatives in desserts revolves around creativity, ingredient selection, portion control, and mindful enjoyment. By embracing these principles, individuals can indulge in delicious treats while supporting their overall health and well-being. Balancing the pleasure of occasional indulgence with nutritious choices can transform dessert time into a guilt-free and satisfying experience.

CHAPTER 11
Meal Plans And Customization

Meal planning is a critical aspect of maintaining a healthy diet, especially for individuals with specific dietary needs or those recovering from health conditions. Weekly meal plans play a pivotal role in ensuring that individuals consume a balanced and nutritious diet consistently.

These plans can be customized to meet various dietary needs, including those of individuals with specific health conditions. Customization involves tailoring meal plans to suit the nutritional requirements, taste preferences, and lifestyle of individual patients. Additionally, meal prep strategies are essential for convenience, ensuring that meals are prepared efficiently and can be easily accessed throughout the week.

Weekly meal plans are structured guides that outline the meals and snacks for each day of the week.

They typically include breakfast, lunch, dinner, and snacks, with an emphasis on incorporating a variety of foods to ensure nutritional adequacy.

For individuals with different dietary needs, such as those following a vegetarian or vegan diet, meal plans can be adjusted to include plant-based protein sources like legumes, tofu, and tempeh. Similarly, individuals following a low-carbohydrate or ketogenic diet may have meal plans that prioritize healthy fats, lean proteins, and non-starchy vegetables while minimizing high-carb foods.

Customizing meal plans for individual patients is essential for addressing their specific health concerns and dietary preferences. This customization can be based on various factors, including age, gender, activity level, food allergies or intolerances, and medical conditions.

For example, a meal plan for a diabetic patient may focus on controlling blood sugar levels through balanced carbohydrate intake, portion control, and choosing low-glycemic index foods.

On the other hand, a meal plan for someone with celiac disease would eliminate gluten-containing grains like wheat, barley, and rye, opting for gluten-free alternatives such as quinoa, brown rice, and certified gluten-free oats.

When creating customized meal plans, healthcare professionals consider the nutritional needs of individual patients. This may involve calculating calorie and macronutrient requirements based on factors like basal metabolic rate, activity level, and weight management goals.

Nutrient-dense foods rich in vitamins, minerals, antioxidants, and fiber are prioritized to support overall health and well-being. Furthermore, meal plans can be adjusted over time based on changes in health status, treatment protocols, or personal preferences.

Meal prep strategies are integral to the success of weekly meal plans, especially for busy individuals or those with limited time for cooking.

Batch cooking, where large quantities of meals are prepared in advance and portioned for later consumption, is a popular meal prep technique. This allows individuals to have ready-to-eat meals throughout the week, reducing the temptation to opt for unhealthy fast food or convenience meals. Using meal prep containers or freezer-friendly dishes can help maintain food quality and freshness.

Another meal prep strategy is ingredient prepping, where key ingredients like chopped vegetables, cooked grains, and marinated proteins are prepared ahead of time. This makes assembling meals quicker and easier during busy weekdays. Additionally, having a well-organized pantry, stocked with essential staples like whole grains, canned beans, nuts, seeds, and healthy cooking oils, streamlines the meal prep process and ensures that nutritious ingredients are readily available.

Incorporating diverse cooking methods, such as baking, grilling, steaming, and sautéing, adds variety to meals and enhances flavor without relying on excessive salt, sugar, or unhealthy fats. Utilizing herbs, spices, citrus juices, and homemade sauces or dressings can elevate the taste of dishes while keeping them nutrient-rich. Moreover, incorporating meal prep into weekly routines fosters a habit of mindful eating, as individuals are more likely to consume balanced meals when they are readily accessible and visually appealing.

Overall, meal plans tailored to different dietary needs, customized for individual patients, and supported by efficient meal prep strategies are key components of a successful nutrition regimen.

By emphasizing variety, nutrient density, and convenience, these approaches empower individuals to make healthier food choices, manage health conditions effectively, and sustain long-term dietary habits that promote well-being.

Conclusion

Cryptosporidiosis recovery hinges on understanding the condition and adopting a tailored nutritional approach. Essential nutrients like lean proteins, healing grains, and immune-boosting ingredients are crucial.

Energizing breakfasts, wholesome mains, and nutrient-rich salads form the foundation. Nourishing soups, brain-boosting beverages, and quick meals offer practical solutions.

Knowing forbidden foods and their substitutes aids in safe eating. Desserts in moderation and customizable meal plans round off a holistic recovery strategy tailored to individual needs.